Alkaline 1

Breakfast Recipes

Insanely Good Alkaline Plant-Based Recipes for Weight Loss & Healing

By Marta Tuchowska
Holistic Wellness Project LTD
Copyright ©Marta Tuchowska 2015, 2016

www.HolisticWellnessProject.com
www.amazon.com/author/mtuchowska

Table of Contents

The Alkaline Diet Lifestyle Cookbook Vol.1

Introduction

Welcome to *The Alkaline Diet Cookbook Part 1* where it's all about healthy and nutritious alkaline diet breakfast recipes that are easy to prepare and will give you the energy you deserve. They will also help you understand the basics of the alkaline diet and lifestyle - even if you have never heard about Alkalinity before. It's focused on keeping things as simple and practical as possible.

This book is for you if:
-you feel like you want to have more energy for life
-you want to learn healthy cooking but don't know where to start
-you are vegan/vegetarian and want to "alkalyze" your way of eating
-you are looking for a natural way to lose weight while giving your body the nutrition it needs
-you want to reduce/eliminate the intake of animal products but don't know how to create recipes that you actually enjoy
-you want to transition towards a natural, wholesome, plant-based, anti-inflammatory diet
-you don't want to spend hours in the kitchen yet want to be able to conjure up healthy and delicious meals that support your health and wellness goals

The Alkaline Diet- The Common Sense Approach

The alkaline diet is a lifestyle that encourages you to give your body the nourishment it needs so that it can work for you at its optimal levels without feeling too exhausted or too acidic. Too much acidity in the body is leading to depression, sickness, and obesity.

Dr. Robert O' Young, Director of Research at the pH Miracle Living Center, says that your fat may be protecting your very life against the acidity in your body. He goes on to make this bold statement.

"There is only one disease: The Constant Acidification of the Body."

What this means is that every disease, including excess weight, is because of a body that is too acidic. These things can make your body too acidic: processed foods, sugar, foods containing gluten and yeast, meat and animal products, stress, alcohol, tobacco, drugs, caffeine, and pollution.

Luckily, the alkaline diet gives us natural tools to fix the problem. I am not talking about overpriced superfoods from overseas that are difficult to find and to pronounce. The simplest methods are always the best and you will be surprised by how healthy you will feel by adding more everyday healing, alkaline foods into your diet (even if you don't follow a strict alkaline diet).

If you attend the root cause of the problem, by implementing a lifestyle rich in alkaline forming foods, it will naturally take care of what plagues you.

My editor, Claire, is a 41-year-old professional woman and a single mom of 3 who suffered from obesity for many years. She just did not have the time to commit to a complicated weight loss program. She made many poor food choices because she was always pressed for time. As a result of her overly acidic body, she experienced tremendous pain from gastric reflux, so much so that her doctor wanted to operate on her.

But once she started following an alkaline plant-based diet (clean, moderate alkaline diet, nothing too strict), she stopped having gastric reflux pain. She began losing weight, and all without feeling deprived and without overdoing or overthinking it. She found she had more energy to get more done each day.

Here are a few simple guidelines that will help you transition towards a healthy, alkaline lifestyle. These are compatible with different nutritional lifestyles (Gluten Free, Vegetarian, Vegan) and it's totally up to you what you choose to focus on:

1) **Eliminate processed foods from your diet and say "no" to colas and sodas** - there are so many additives and preservatives in these foods. They have been known to create hormone imbalances, make you tired, and add to acidity in your body. It's just not natural for humans to consume those conveniently processed foods. The label may even say "low in calories or low in fat"- it will not help you in your long term weight loss or health efforts. In order to start losing weight naturally, your body needs foods that are jam-packed with nutrients. Real foods. Living foods. This, in turn, will help your body maintain its optimal blood pH (7.35) almost effortlessly.

2) **Add more raw foods into your diet**- especially lots of vegetables and leafy greens as well as fruits that are naturally low in sugar (for example, limes, lemons, grapefruits, avocados, tomatoes, and pomegranates are alkaline forming fruits).

3) **Reduce/eliminate animal products** – these are extremely acid-forming. The good news is that there are many plant-based options out there and tons of way to create delicious alkaline-friendly plant-based meals you will love! If I could do it, you can do it too.

4) **Drink plenty of clean, filtered water**, preferably alkaline water or fruit-infused water.

5) **Add more vegetable juices into your diet**- these are a great way to give your body more nutrients and alkalinity that will result in more energy, less inflammation and, if desired- natural weight loss. Vegetable juices are the best shots of health! I have also

written a book called: "Alkaline Juicing" if want to give it a try and want to juice the right way.

6) **Reduce/eliminate processed grains, "crappy carbs" as well as yeast** (very acid-forming). Personally, I recommend quinoa instead (it's naturally gluten-free), amaranth (very nutritious), brown rice, or soba noodles (it's made from buckwheat and naturally gluten-free). You can also use gluten-free wraps or make your own bread. Fruit is also a great natural source of carbohydrates, and great for energy. Plus, they always make a great snack!

7) **Reduce/eliminate caffeine**- trust me - it will only make you feel sick and tired in the long run, and can even lead to adrenal exhaustion (not the best condition to end up in - I have been there). It may seem a bit drastic at first, and yes, I know what you're thinking- there are so many articles out there praising benefits of caffeine and coffee. Yes, I am sure there are, as many people build their business around coffee. This is why there must be something out there that promotes it. At the same time, I agree that everything is good for you in moderation. As long as you have a healthy foundation, you can have coffee as a treat (I do drink coffee occasionally). There is no reason to be too strict on yourself. But...don't rely on caffeine as your main source of energy. Green tea may be helpful too as a transition, but green tea is not caffeine-free either so don't overdo it. On the other side of spectrum - green tea is rich in antioxidants and a great part of a balanced diet, so it's not that you have to get paranoid about all kinds of caffeine. Moderation is the key. Try to observe your body. Personally, I have noticed that quitting my

coffee habits (I used to have 2-3 coffees a day) and replacing coffee with natural herbal teas and infusions have really made my energy levels skyrocket. Now I sleep better, and I get up feeling nice and fresh. I don't need caffeine to keep me awake. I no longer suffer from tension headaches and I feel calmer. Yes, I do have a cup of coffee as a treat sometimes, usually when I meet with a friend, but I no longer depend on it. I choose it; it doesn't choose me. Think about this and how you can apply this simple tip to your life to achieve total wellbeing. Coffee and caffeine in general is extremely acid-forming.

I recently started using an Ayurvedic herb called Ashwagandha. It is known as an adaptogenic herb and it can help you restore your energy levels naturally. I highly recommend you give it a try!

8) **Replace cow's milk with almond milk, coconut milk or any other vegan friendly milk** (for example quinoa milk, chia seed milk, oats milk- whatever works for you and your stomach) that works well for you. Cow's milk is extremely acid forming and personally, I don't think it makes sense for humans to drink milk that is naturally designed for fattening baby calves not humans. Actually, quitting dairy was one of the best things I have done for myself. I have noticed that even very little milk would cause digestive problems and it was really easy to fix-I quit drinking milk. I also learned about cruelty in the dairy industry which obviously contributed to my decision. The best thing about the alkaline plant-based diet is that you can still have ice cream and other treats- you just make them with no milk/animal products. It's so much healthier and tastier, totally guilt-free. With this

approach, there is no need to go hungry or deprived. You focus on abundance of foods and meals that are good for you, delicious and such a choice is also better for the animals and the planet. This is what I call- holistic motivation.

9) **Don't fear good fats- coconut oil, olive oil, avocado oil** etc. are good for you and should replace processed margarines, and artery-clogging trans-fats. This is not to say that you can "drink" them freely. Balance is the key.

Also...

Use stevia instead of processed sugar (stevia is sweet but sugar-free) and Himalayan salt instead of regular salt (Himalayan salt contain some amounts of calcium, iron, potassium and magnesium plus it also contains lower amounts of sodium than regular salt.)

Add more spices and herbs into your diet- not only do they make your dishes taste amazing but they also have anti-inflammatory properties and help you detoxify (cilantro, turmeric, and cinnamon are miraculous).

As you can see, the alkaline diet is a pretty common sense clean diet. Nothing is exaggerated. Nothing is too strict. Nothing is too faddish. Eat more living foods and avoid processed foods. Try to eat more plant based foods. Don't reject it before you have tried it.

Add regular relaxation techniques to the alkaline diet (including yoga, meditation), time spent in nature, adequate sleep and physical activity (we need to sweat out those toxins) and you have a prescription for health. It's strange to me that there are so many people putting the alkaline diet down, however, the general guidelines I have mentioned above are common sense for a healthy lifestyle and I am sure your doctor would agree with it (more natural foods, less processed crap, more relaxation, less stress). This is the gist of the alkaline diet lifestyle. This is what will make you feel nice and rejuvenated and achieve your ideal weight. The problem is that some people are not willing to take those small common sense steps and are looking for a "secret formula" something that will magically help them with no effort at all. I am not judging- I have been guilty of it as well. We all have!

The truth is that whatever changes you want to make in your life (this rule applies not only to health) can be hard as leaving one's comfort zone is difficult, but with time and practise it becomes easy and automatic. Holistic success is about applying what we already know and using the information to better our lives. This is what I call "the secret formula." Information in action.

I always say that I am very open-minded when it comes to different diets. I never claim that what I do is the only path to wellness and health. I prefer to provide you with information and inspiration so that you can create your own way and choose what works for you. Everyone is different. What I teach is based on the alkaline way of living I learned from Doctor Young. However, my alkaline diet may be a bit different than yours and we can still be doing it the right way.

You need to learn to listen to your body and be good on yourself.

Now, with that being said, simply try to adhere to the following recommendations - they will help you understand the gist of the alkaline diet without overwhelming you with complicated pH discussions.

You can easily get started today- simply by making some minor adjustments to your existing diet. Baby steps. I always try to make things simple and easy to apply. Once you apply it - you will feel the amazing benefits of Alkalinity and from there you will want to carry on.

The alkaline diet is not a diet but a lifestyle really. It encourages you to add more alkalizing foods and drinks into your diet so that your body can heal itself naturally. How?

Alkaline Diet Crash Course- Understand the Basics

The pH of most of our important cellular and other fluids (like blood) is actually designed to be at pH of 7.35 (slightly alkaline).

The body has an intricate system in place to always maintain that healthy, slightly alkaline pH level – no matter what you eat. This is an argument that many alkaline diet skeptics use and I get it. It's 100% true.

This is not the goal of the alkaline diet. We just can't make our blood's pH more alkaline or "higher." Our body tries to work really hard for us to help us maintain our ideal pH (7.35). We can't have a pH of 8 or 9. If we did we would be dead.

The entire focus of the alkaline diet is to give your body the nourishment and healing tools it needs to MAINTAIN that optimal 7.35 pH almost effortlessly.

If we fail to do so, we torture our body with an incredible stress! Yes- when the body has to constantly work overtime to detoxify all the cells and maintain our pH it finally succumbs to disease.

Let me just name a few cases of what can happen if we constantly eat an acid-forming diet (also called SAD - Standard American Diet) that is not supporting our body at all. Our body ends up sick and tired of working overtime and may manifest one or more of the following conditions:

-constant inflammation

-immune and hormone imbalance

-lack of energy, mental fog

-yeast and candida overgrowth

-digestive damage

-weakened bones (our body is forced to pull minerals like magnesium and calcium from our bones in order to maintain alkaline balance it needs for constant healing processes).

In summary, eating more alkaline foods helps support our body so that it can work for us at optimal levels while eating more acidic food doesn't help at all. The alkaline diet is not about magically raising our pH but helping our body rebalance itself by supporting its natural healing functions.

However, it's not only about what we eat - it's also about how we live and what we think. It's not just a diet; it's a lifestyle. If you want vibrant health and alkaline wellness, try to be outdoors more, meditate, laugh, spend time with family and friends, do things you enjoy so that you can de-stress, practise mindfulness...It's not only about nutrition.

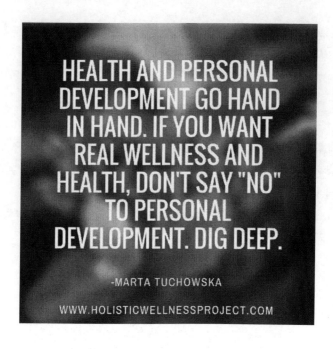

HEALTH AND PERSONAL
DEVELOPMENT GO HAND
IN HAND. IF YOU WANT
REAL WELLNESS AND
HEALTH, DON'T SAY "NO"
TO PERSONAL
DEVELOPMENT. DIG DEEP.

-MARTA TUCHOWSKA

WWW.HOLISTICWELLNESSPROJECT.COM

Over the years, I have also learned that obsessing too much about food or health can be bad. You see - when you are too strict on yourself, this attitude takes away your emotional wellness. Balance is the key: we don't want to be too strict and too obsessed, but we don't want to end up being too lenient as well. You need to be honest with yourself and ask yourself what you can do better and reclaim responsibility for your health and wellness. It's always great to look for that next level, however it's also good to cultivate the sense of gratitude and accomplishment for what we have already managed to change in our diets and lifestyles. Keep learning new recipes and gaining more information about alkaline/vegan/plant based lifestyles. Just keep moving forward, you will get there. Trying is winning!

Oftentimes, it's not about eating less - but about eating right.

Your Free Gifts + Free Alkaline Newsletter

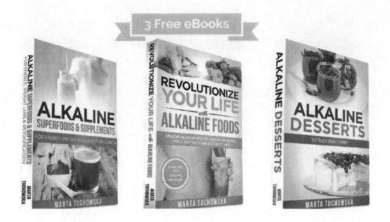

Never heard of the Alkaline Diet and don't know where to start?

I remember when I first learned about the alkaline diet. I was more than confused and sceptical. I wanted to take action but didn't know how. I would spend endless hours online looking for alkaline-acid charts only to find there was way too much contradictory information out there.

I don't want you to feel confused. I also really appreciate the fact you took an interest in my work. This is why I would love to offer you 3 free alkaline diet & lifestyle eBooks + **easy alkaline-acid charts** (printable so that you can keep them on your fridge or in your wallet). They will provide a solid foundation to kick-start your alkaline diet success. You will get all the facts explained in plain English, practical alkaline tips, and yummy, vegan-friendly recipes full of taste, motivational advice, as well as printable charts for quick reference.

Visit:

www.HolisticWellnessProject.com/alkaline

to grab them now!

If you happen to have any problems, write us at:

info@holisticwellnessproject.com

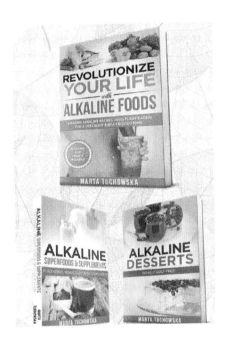

The benefits of eating more alkaline & plant-based foods

Since animal products are acid-forming, the alkaline diet is pretty vegan and plant-based in its design. I always try to encourage people to try to stick with vegan options as much as possible- it's fun, it's creative and much more sustainable and better for our environment. Veganism and alkalinity very often overlap and many "alkalarians" are vegans or vegetarians, but we need to remember that vegans stick to their choices not only for their own health, but they also act against animal cruelty and climate changes. People go vegan for a variety of reasons including both their own health, environment, love for animals, even spiritual reasons etc. I believe that an alkaline diet can be a great stepping stone towards veganism.

This is what it did for me; first I reduced animal products, then I decided to go vegetarian (no meat) and finally, a few months ago, I decided to go fully vegan (no animal products whatsoever) and I am loving this lifestyle. I wish I had started it earlier (I lacked information and did not have the right mindset). When I first began my alkaline journey, my own health was my main motivation. I suffered from a really rare eye disease triggered by inflammation and auto-immune system disorders and going alkaline has helped me with my treatment. This is how I became really passionate about it. I finally reached the "almost vegan" stage of my diet and in March 2016, after researching tons of information on veganism, educating myself and learning all the cruelty in the meat and dairy industry, I made a decision to go fully vegan. As you can see, in my case it was a process. I don't mean to be judgemental, do "holier than thou" or tell people that my way is better than theirs, but since I am experiencing all the fantastic benefits of this alkaline-vegan lifestyle, I want to share this information with as many people as I can.

To sum up - if you can't imagine yourself going vegan at this point, that's fine. Simply try to enrich your diet with more alkaline, plant-based options reducing animal products at the same time. This book will give you dozens of ideas to make a transition a really enjoyable experience. It's not very hard and you will feel healthier and energized as you eat more alkaline and less acid-forming. With the recipes you are just about to discover, I can guarantee that you won't feel deprived or bored. Having plenty of proven recipes is the key to success and the more you learn, the more motivated you will feel.

We also need to keep in mind that the alkaline diet is not about eating 100% alkaline or fully raw. It's not about surviving on cucumbers and kale. Simply try to make about 70% of your diet rich in alkaline-forming foods, it's as simple as that. Whenever in doubt, please check the charts that come as an additional, free resource with this book. You can download and print them at:
www.holisticwellnessproject.com/alkaline

You may want to keep them at hand while shopping, or even going through my recipes.

About the recipes:

- Most ingredients are really easy, everyday and "common sense" ingredients that are easy to find at your local grocery store or supermarket. Occasionally, I may give you some recommendations for natural food supplements or some unusual super foods, but these are not the only path to wellness. The reason why I mention them is for informative purposes, in case you wish to add some new stuff into your diet or you simply like experimenting. Many of those "rare superfood" ingredients can be ordered on-line from Amazon.

- You don't need to be a good cook or a qualified chef to learn those simple and delicious recipes. Honestly, I have never been "spend all her free time in her kitchen" girl (of course there is nothing wrong with that if you are absolutely passionate about cooking, but most people are too tired or too pressed for time). While I do enjoy cooking, as I am attracted to the *creative* part of it as well as health benefits that I can rip off if I cook the right way, I always try to make the whole process as simple as possible. I am a big fan of automation as well and so I like batch-cooking to make sure I always have some healthy options to fall, back on. Let's be real - everyone can have a bad day and cooking may seem like a mission. This is why having something that is already waiting for you that you prepared in advance is a great life saver. This is especially true if you are on a busy schedule or have a big family to feed.

- You don't need any fancy kitchen equipment to get started on my recipes. While having a good blender or food processor helps and so does food spiralizer, you can also use a simple hand blender and a knife. Add to it chopping boards, oven, pans and pots and you have all you need.

- Most of my recipes are quick to prepare- give it 20 minutes or less and you have a delicious and nutritious meal that supports your health and fitness goals.

Again, let's remember that the alkaline diet is not about eating 100% alkaline. Let's aim for 70%. It's so much easier, right? The remaining 30% can be acidic foods, but this not justify processed foods that need to be buried forever. Your number one goal should be to eliminate all processed convenience foods. Then keep trying different foods and recipes and observe what works for you.

I always say that you need to listen to your body. On top of that, any drastic changes in your diet should be discussed with your doctor.

The Alkaline Diet Made Easy. Even for Busy People

As soon as you try my recipes and eat more alkaline, you will soon start noticing all the benefits of eating a diet jam-packed with vitamins, minerals, natural protein, fibre, healthy fats as well as free of artificial sugar, gluten and other processed foods.

Now, here's why many people fail with the alkaline diet and healthy eating in general. I am not judging as I have been guilty of it many times. It stems from the fact that a person gets passionate about health, but tries to do it all at once or doesn't know where to start. You need a good strategy to fall back on.

It's simple, if you only rely on willpower your goals probably are:
-just ignore all the cravings and hold on
-eat only healthy alkaline foods and be strong and stick to it- if I have to survive on salads so be it!

Unfortunately, this strategy is not a plan I recommend. It may not last for too long unless you are a super strong-willed person.

Here's the problem with this approach and I have faced it so many times:

You end up eating the same stuff all the time, and you get obsessed about foods. So you stress too much about the whole healthy eating thing. It means that you are constantly wondering what you're going to eat or what you just ate. Anxiety and guilt trips form part of this self-torture and it seems like health and wellness success is farther and farther away.

Then you think about your family and friends. They think you're a rabbit! They eat some yummy stuff and you are right in front of them with another boring salad (let me guess- iceberg lettuce, tomatoes and cucumber?).

It's not hard to fail in this scenario. In fact it's pretty normal. It would be weird if you didn't fail while following this crazy strategy. The risks could be that you don't get proper nutrition you need (you just worry too much about your pH) and your emotional wellness just leaves you.

The good news is that Marta is here to show you how to do it right with her recipes so that you eat a clean, balanced plant-based diet inspired by the alkaline diet and compatible with your current nutritional lifestyle. You enjoy it and so it's not that hard for you to create a healthy lifestyle. Moreover, it's cool to get new skills in the kitchen and treat your family and friends to healthy and delicious meals.

Alkaline Diet- Common Questions

Are lemons acidic or alkaline?
This is my favourite question and if you are a beginner, it's normal you are asking it. The answer is very simple: it's all about the effect that the food has on our body after it has been consumed, not before. It doesn't matter to us what pH they have in their natural state (before they have been eaten). Lemons are full of alkaline minerals and at the same time they don't contain sugar which makes them one of the very few alkaline fruits.
Remember to get your starter's guide and food list at:
www.holisticwellnessproject.com/alkaline
They will save you confusion.

What about Protein?
The choice to avoid/reduce the consumption of meat and other animal-derived products is becoming increasingly accepted among the general public. Restaurants and supermarkets are catering for vegans and those opting for an alkaline diet ever more than in the past offering a wide selection of delicious and vegan-friendly products. Some of these foods have been crafted to imitate certain things that you may wish to continue to enjoy, just in a novel, plant-based

form, instead. Such things include non-dairy ice cream and yogurt, for example. Other foods, of course, are naturally vegan-friendly with even their conventional forms being entirely of plant origin.

Although the issue of finding vegan-friendly, alkaline products and restaurant items is becoming less of a problem in big cities and healthy food stores, this does not mean that this availability translates into a simple and easy life of making everyday vegan dishes at home. It's this particular challenge that we are now going to tackle with the help of the book you now hold in your hands. Making tasty and nutritious alkaline friendly dishes at home doesn't need to be difficult or expensive, and you'll soon be able to use the recipes in this book to prove it to yourself once and for all.

Plant-based protein:
- Hemp (You can use hemp powder in your smoothies.)
- Green leafy veggies (One cup of cooked spinach has about 7 grams of protein. Kale is pretty much the same.)
- Quinoa (It has about 9 grams of protein per cup.)
- Almond Butter (It is great with gluten-free breads and wraps. Two tablespoons of almond butter is about 8 grams of protein.)
- Other choices include: lentils (great in salads), beans and chickpeas
- Nuts and seeds (for example sunflower seeds)

HEALTH BENEFITS OF VEGAN/ALKALINE/PLANT-BASED DIETS:
- lower cholesterol levels
-lower blood pressure,

-lower rates of Type 2 diabetes,
-lower risk of death from heart disease,
-lower overall cancer rates
-less acidity in the body
-natural weight loss
-clean skin
-healthier immune system
-improved digestion

Recommended resources:
www.nutritionfacts.org by Doctor Michael Greger.
His website offers tons of great information as well as
scientifically proven approach to plant based diets.

Do I have to give up my favourite foods forever?

Luckily, you don't. The mere thought of having to give
everything up is just unbearable, right? Don't try to be perfect.
Focus on progress. For example, in my opinion, people do
much better if they try to be 70-80% great and 20-30% relaxed
than if they try to be 100% perfect- all the time. This rule also
applies to other goals, not only health. This approach is so
much easier when you are just starting out!

It is also important to remember that you can still have your
favorite foods (ice cream, pizzas, even burgers) in their vegan,
alkaline versions! This is great news! Again, it's not that you
have to survive on green smoothies alone.

Besides, if you try to be perfect (for example, you try to stick
100% to smoothies and salads) you may experience many

negative emotions (deprivation) that are not healthy. In fact, stressing too much about food or life in general, can be very acid-forming.

Now it's not a secret that raw foods are more alkaline than cooked foods. But you can still be alkaline even if you don't follow a 100% raw food diet (you can if you want to, but it's not the only path to wellness and health). Personally, my number one rule is to keep it all plant based, and 70-80% alkaline. I also like combining cooked foods with raw foods. My body tells me what's good for me and my digestion.

You don't have to give up your life. You can still go out with friends and socialize. You can still have that glass of wine or an occasional coffee.

Alcohol is highly acid-forming, but you can enjoy a couple of drinks on social occasions every now and then. I am not talking about getting drunk of course, but there is nothing wrong with having an occasional drink with a friend and having a laugh. The problem is when you feel you need a drink because you can't deal with stress or you need it to boost your confidence (I have been there, I am not judging). In that case, I recommend you resort to meditation, hypnosis, NLP, yoga, natural remedies, and guided meditation. You can download a free audiobook I created for you at:

www.HolisticWellnessProject.com/mindfulness

There are many options out there that can help you create a new, stronger, more stress-free and more confident version of yourself with long-term success.

So back to acid-forming foods and drinks, just remember-moderation is the key. It's not that you will have to give up all the acidic foods forever. At the same time, I am not saying you should be indulging in unhealthy foods all the time. Just follow your own pace.

However, I strongly recommend you give up sodas and other artificial drinks as well as chemically processed foods, and convenience foods. They do not bring you closer to your goals at all. There are healthier snacks out there, you can make your own fries and crisps, and you can experiment with fruit infused water that is a great alternative to sodas and also much, much cheaper.

Also don't try to do it all at once. Set simple goals. For example: this week I will replace sodas with fruit infused water. Action plan: get the recipes and ingredients. Done? Great. Next step. Repeat the process, for example: this week I will try to drink one alkaline smoothie a day and have some salad with my lunch/dinner. Done? Great. Create the next step. For example: this week, I will get committed to physical activity or yoga. Only one step at the time. Baby steps. Here and now. I call it- mindful motivation.

Now, with all of that information out of the way, it's time to start looking at some delicious recipes. Each category includes a number of tasty dishes with a little description telling you what's so good about it from a nutritional/lifestyle point of view. You'll also find easy to follow instructions for each dish, so you'll never have a moment's hesitation when making beautiful and healthy dishes for you and your loved ones.

Shall you happen to have any questions or doubts about this book (or you want to say hi) just email me at:
info@holisticwellnessproject.com
I love hearing from my readers!

Important:
I am not a doctor/therapist or a scientist, and I am not giving you any specific advice related to serious health problems. So if you happen to have any specific health questions, remember to talk to your doctor or health professional first. Please read a full disclaimer at the beginning of this book.

As a wellness coach I help people with **motivation**, habits and **practical holistic self-care tips** so that they can create a healthy lifestyle with long-term benefits that allows them to prevent numerous illnesses and lose weight in a healthy way. I call it a holistic lifestyle design, something that I am absolutely passionate about and honestly, I am even more passionate about helping you being passionate about it as well. This is my mission and this is what I stand for. I want to help you work on your body, mind and soul so that you can create success in all areas of life. It all starts with energy and vibrant health.

Also, remember that you can also use my recipes as templates to create your own. If there is any ingredient you don't like or your body can't tolerate - skip it. We need to listen to our body and be selective if necessary. Everyone is different and so are their nutritional preferences. Follow your way (but try to keep it plant based as much as you can, sorry I had to make this remark).

Read on and enjoy!

Don't forget to download your free complimentary eBooks at: www.holisticwellnessproject.com/alkaline

Recipe Measurements

I love keeping ingredient measurements as simple as possible-this is why I stick to tablespoons, teaspoons and cups.
The cup measurement I use is the American cup measurement. I also use it for dry ingredients. If you are new to it, let me help you:
If you don't have American Cup measures, just use a metric or imperial liquid measuring jug and fill your jug with your ingredient to the corresponding level. Here's how to go about it:
1 American Cup= 250ml= 8 fl.oz

For example:
If a recipe calls for 1 cup of almonds, simply place your almonds into your measuring jug until it reaches the 250 ml/8oz mark.
I know that different countries use different measurements and I wanted to make things simple for you.

# Translations (US-UK English)
Eggplant=Aubergine
Zucchini=Courgette
Cilantro=Coriander
Garbanzo Beans=Chickpeas
Navy Beans-=Haricot Beans
Aragula=Rocket
Broth=Stock

Beautiful Alkaline-Diet-Inspired Clean Eating Breakfasts

Breakfast can be one of the biggest challenges for new "alkalarians" as well as many people who want to get healthy. It may also be hard to adapt breakfasts if you have no idea how to make them both nice and quick as well as delicious and nutritious. However, it doesn't have to be this way. You are just about to discover that you have another option. Say goodbye to heavy breakfasts that are way difficult to digest and forget about skipping breakfasts with a cup of coffee (coffee is acid-forming, while it's OK as a little treat every now and then, it should not be abused).

It's not about eating less or going hungry, it's about eating right. You can enjoy a wide variety of clean meals composed of plenty of healing alkaline foods which will give you that morning boost you so desperately need. The recipes below are meant to give you an idea of the delicious, and yet simple, creations you can make every morning to fill your body with goodness so that it is ready for the day ahead.

Give yourself the energy you deserve first thing in the morning. If you start your day healthy, you will end your day feeling healthy! Whether you wake up craving sweetness or are planning to do some healthy baking to create some nice and guilt-free breakfast treats these recipes will give you both. If you need to have a solid breakfast because you wake up hungry, or are looking for a quick breakfast snack, raw food options or a takeaway breakfast you are about to discover a myriad of alkaline-friendly, clean diet recipes to pick and choose from depending on your mood and taste preferences. Choosing what you want to eat will make you feel better about eating a healthy, nutritious breakfast in the morning.

This is not a book on strict dieting, but a book on creating a healthy and balanced lifestyle through alkaline food inspired nutrition. My goal is to help you achieve long term success and help you spare frustration, fad diets and stress that you may experience when counting calories.

SECTION I
Porridges, Puddings, Pancakes, Bakes

Almost Alkaline Choco Porridge

Although chocolate doesn't sound like much of a breakfast, pure cocoa contains an extraordinarily high level of antioxidants and beneficial plant fats. We won't be using the typical chocolate you're thinking of; the one devoid of all nutrition. You can use cocoa powder to get all the beneficial effects of the delicious cocoa bean. Combined with almonds and quinoa, this recipe makes for a perfectly energy-dense morning boost. It is great for mental focus and concentration. Raw cocoa is not super alkaline, however this recipes balances it with more alkaline ingredients to create a super powerful breakfast for busy people. Yum!

Serves: 2
Ingredients:
- Half cup cooked quinoa
- 2 tbsp. raw cocoa powder, unsweetened
- 2 cups almond or coconut milk
- Handful of almonds, chopped
- Handful of dried cranberries or other fruit of your choice
- 2 tbsp. desiccated coconut
- 2 tbsp. raw almond butter, unsweetened
- 1 tbsp. ginger powder

Optional:
- 2 tbsp. barley grass powder for more alkaline benefits and nutrition

- 2 tbsp. chia seeds for more nutrition

Instructions:

1. Mix the quinoa and unsweetened cocoa powder in a breakfast cereal bowl(s).
2. Pour the coconut milk (or other plant-derived milk) into the bowl and mix well. If the mixture is too dry, add a little more.
3. It's best to cover this mixture and allow it to sit overnight. You don't have to do this if you would prefer not to, though.
4. Stir the mixture and then add the ginger powder, almonds and cranberries and other fruit of your choice.
5. Scatter the desiccated coconut over the top of the mixture and place the almond butter in the middle.
6. Give it all a quick stir and enjoy.

Alka Paleo Flax Seed Mix

Great option for breakfast on the go. It's all too common to run out the door without eating anything, but as soon as we do it, we end up grabbing whatever is available, and *not* making the best choices. Here is one of my favorites; simply blend all together and enjoy!

Serves: 2
Ingredients:
- 2 avocados, peeled, pitted and chopped
- 1 cup almond milk or coconut milk
- 1 tablespoon ground flax seeds (chia could work great here, too)
- ½ cup soy sprouts (I am not talking about soy, but soy sprouts)
- Olive oil and Himalayan salt to taste

Instructions:
Blend and enjoy!

Alkaline Panna Cotta

Panna Cotta is a traditional Italian dessert recipe that also makes a great breakfast meal. I was able to transform this recipe and make it dairy-free and vegan/alkaline friendly. If you want to enjoy it for breakfast, you will need to get into a habit of preparing it after dinner and let it form properly overnight. It will only take a few minutes to prepare and trust me - it will be easier for you to wake up and get up knowing that there is an amazing panna cotta waiting for you.

Serves: 2-3
Ingredients:
- 1 cup coconut milk
- 1 cup almond milk (unsweetened) - if you are allergic to almond, use coconut milk or organic rice milk instead (total 2 cups, if you want to use more milk, use more gelatin as well)
- 2 tablespoons of unflavored vegan-friendly Gelatin (Unflavored Vegan Gel)
- 2 tablespoons Stevia
- 2 teaspoons vanilla extract
- 2 teaspoons cinnamon powder
- Juice of 1 lemon
- 2 tablespoons chia seeds
- OPTIONAL: 2 TABLESPOONS BARLEY GRASS (it's jam-packed with nutrients)
- Toppings of your choice (maybe homemade marmalade or some fruit?)

Instructions:
1. Pour the milk mix into a saucepan and add in gelatin.
2. Whisk steadily for 5 minutes (no heat).

3. Then, add in stevia, cinnamon, vanilla, chia seeds and green powders (this is optional).
4. Turn on the heat (medium heat) and keep stirring constantly, until milk is hot enough to steam.
5. Important- Do not boil as this will deactivate the gelling properties of the gelatin.
6. Turn off the heat and leave to cool down for a few minutes.
7. In the meantime, grease small bowls with coconut oil and pour the heated mixture into the bowls.
8. Cover and place in the fridge for about 8 hours (yep...you have to wait 8 hours...that's the only drawback of this recipe)
9. When ready, serve directly in bowls (like I did here, nothing too artistic really - I was pressed for time) or gently turn them upside down on to a place and add toppings (this is what I am going to do for my special guests!)

Awesome Energy Bars

Great recipe for batch-cooking to make sure you always have a ready to grab healthy breakfast option!

Makes 5-6 bars
Ingredients:
- 1 banana, mashed
- 1/4 cup almonds
- 1/3 cup dried plums
- 1/4 cup sunflower seeds
- 1/4 cup vanilla or hemp protein powder
- 2 tbsp. arrowroot starch
- 1/2 cup almond flour

Instructions:
1. Combine mashed banana with almond flour and arrowroot starch.
2. Mix well and then add in dried plums, nuts, seeds, almond flour and protein powder. Place through a food processor.
3. Add mix to a pan greased with coconut oil and bake at 275 °F (130 °C) for about 30 minutes.
4. Remove and let cool then cut into bars or squares.
5. Enjoy!

Cinnamon Quinoa Bowl

Servings: 2
Ingredients:
- 1 cup uncooked quinoa
- 1 ½ cups water
- ½ teaspoon ground cinnamon
- Pinch of Himalayan salt

Instructions:
1. Rinse the quinoa well.
2. In a medium-sized saucepan, combine the quinoa, water, cinnamon and salt.
3. Bring to a boil.
4. Then, turn down the heat, cover, and simmer for 10 minutes.
5. When cooked, remove from the heat.
6. Cool down.
7. Serve drizzled with coconut or almond milk.
8. Enjoy!

Vegan Apple Cinnamon Muffins

Here comes another treat recipe. While alkaline diet tries to avoid sugar in all its forms, it's totally okay to use some stevia for natural sweetness (stevia is not sugar).

Servings: 12
Ingredients:
- 1 ½ tablespoon flaxseed meal
- 2 ½ tablespoons warm water
- 3 teaspoons coconut oil
- 2 large ripe apples, diced
- 1 cup unsweetened coconut milk
- ¾ cup lemon juice
- A few drops of stevia
- 3 tablespoons vegetable oil
- ½ tablespoon vanilla extract
- 1 ½ cups gluten-free flour blend
- 1 ½ teaspoon ground cinnamon
- 1 teaspoon baking soda
- Pinch of Himalayan salt
- ½ cup old-fashioned oats (gluten-free)

Instructions:
1. Preheat your oven to a temperature of 375°F (190 Celsius).
2. Line a muffin pan with paper liners.
3. Using a bowl, whisk the flaxseed and water together. Let rest for 10 minutes.
4. Heat the coconut oil over the medium heat (use a small saucepan)
5. Add the apples and toss them with cinnamon then cook for a few minutes until soft.

42

6. Remove the apples from heat.
7. Combine the almond milk, lemon juice, stevia, oil, and the vanilla extract in a mixing bowl.
8. Whisk in the flax mixture until it is super smooth.
9. In a separate bowl, mix together the gluten-free flour blend, cinnamon, and baking soda as well as Himalayan salt.
10. Mix the dry ingredients with the wet ingredients until smooth.
11. Carefully fold in the oats and the sautéed apples.
12. Place the batter into the prepared muffin pan, filling the cups completely.
13. Bake for about 20 minutes until a knife inserted in the center comes out clean.
14. Cool the muffins for 15-20 minutes, serve and enjoy!

Avocado Choco Mousse

If you like healthy treats for breakfast, be sure to prepare this one before you go to bed. Just like with the panna cotta, it needs some time to sit well.

Servings: 6 to 8
Ingredients:
- 1/2 cup cocoa powder
- 4 large ripe avocados, pitted and chopped
- ½ cup unsweetened almond milk
- 1 tablespoon pure vanilla extract
- A few drops of liquid stevia
- ¼ cup soaked almonds

Instructions:
1. In a blender or food processor, blend the mixture until smooth and well combined.
2. Spoon into dessert cups and chill for 4 to 6 hours before serving.
3. Enjoy!

Vegan Paleo-Friendly Porridge

This recipe is both alkaline and paleo friendly. It offers a highly energizing mix of seeds that is nicely alkalized by spices and lemon juice. It's a perfect breakfast for busy people. No excuses - don't skip breakfast.

Servings: 1
Ingredients:
- ¼ cup chopped walnuts
- 2 tablespoons pumpkin seeds
- 1 tablespoon raw chia seeds
- 1 teaspoon ground cinnamon
- 1 teaspoon nutmeg
- 1 cup almond milk or coconut milk
- 1 tablespoon of melted coconut oil
- Juice of 1 lemon
- Juice of 1 grapefruit
- Optional: 1 teaspoon of barley grass powder

Instructions:
1. Combine your ingredients in a cereal bowl and pour over some coconut or almond milk.
2. Stir well and serve.
3. Enjoy!

Amaranth Coconut Porridge

Amaranth is a great source of iron and of the healthiest of the grains there are. Personally, I prefer quinoa, but I like to switch to amaranth every now and then. Variety is the key. Both quinoa and amaranth are gluten-free and a spectacular addition to a balanced diet.

Servings: 2
Ingredients:
- 2 cups water
- 1 cup amaranth
- 1 cup coconut milk
- ½ cup shredded coconut, slightly toasted

Instructions:
1. Add amaranth to boiling water.
2. Reduce heat and simmer on medium heat for 15- 20 minutes until amaranth is cooked.
3. Remove from heat and stir in the coconut milk as well as the toasted coconut.
4. Add some stevia to sweeten if you wish (you can also serve it with some homemade marmalade) and enjoy!

Cinnamon Pumpkin Porridge

With a variety of porridge recipes in this book, there is no chance you will ever get bored. Here comes another delicious recipe with anti-inflammatory, alkalizing properties.

Servings: 2
Ingredients:
- 1 cup unsweetened almond milk or coconut milk
- 1 cup water
- 1 cup uncooked quinoa
- ½ cup pumpkin puree
- 1 teaspoon ground cinnamon
- 2 tablespoons ground flaxseed meal
- Juice of 1 lemon

Instructions:
1. Whisk together the water and almond milk.
2. Bring the mixture to boil.
3. Stir in the quinoa, pumpkin, and cinnamon.
4. Reduce the heat.
5. Cover and simmer for 10 minutes or until the liquid has been absorbed.
6. Remove from the heat and then stir in the flaxseed meal.
7. Place the porridge into small bowls.
8. Sprinkle some lemon juice and add some pumpkin seeds on top if desired.

Hemp Protein Crepes

Meat is not the only way to get protein, there are many other plant-based options out there and this recipe is the best proof of how you can combine taste and health.

Hemp seed is full of essential fats, antioxidants, amino acids, fiber, iron, zinc, carotene, vitamin B1, vitamin B2, vitamin B6, vitamin D, vitamin E, chlorophyll, calcium, magnesium, copper, potassium, phosphorus, and enzymes just to name a few. If you want to eat more vegan, make sure to add some hemp seeds into your diet.

Servings: 4 to 6
Ingredients:
- 3 cups of almond milk
- 2 tablespoons of coconut oil, melted
- 2 cups rice flour or almond flour
- ¼ cup hemp seeds (raw)
- 1 ripe banana, peeled and mashed
- Olive oil or coconut oil, as needed

Instructions:
1. In a mixing bowl, combine the almond milk, coconut oil, flour, and hemp seeds.
2. Whisk until well combined.
3. Add in the mashed banana – stir until lump-free.
4. Heat some olive oil or coconut oil using a small skillet (medium heat).
5. Pour in about ¼ cup of the batter and tilt the pan to coat the bottom well.
6. Cook for a few minutes or until the edges of the crepe are dry and nicely browned.
7. Flip carefully and cook on the other side.

8. Repeat the process to create more protein pancakes.
9. Enjoy!

Coconut Apple Choco Stir Fry

Craving something sweet? Here comes a perfect guilt-free solution that is also full of nutrition. As you may have noticed, I like barley grass powder a lot. It's full of nutrients and alkalizing properties.

Serves: 2
Ingredients:
- 2 green apples, peeled and chopped
- 1 tablespoons coconut oil
- 1 teaspoon cinnamon powder
- 2 tablespoons chia seeds
- Stevia to sweeten
- 2 tablespoons raw cocoa powder
- 1 tablespoon of barley grass

Instructions:
1. Heat up some coconut oil in a frying pan.
2. Add the apples, cinnamon, stevia and cook until soft.
3. Turn off the heat and add some raw cocoa and chia seeds.
4. Stir well.
5. Place in dessert bowls, sprinkle over some barley grass.
6. Cool down in a fridge, serve and enjoy!

Easy Anti Inflammatory Apple Treat

Sugar and artificial ingredients aggravate inflammation while living foods and spices help alleviate it. If you are looking for yummy breakfast ideas with anti-inflammatory properties this is the recipe for you.

Servings: 4 to 6
Ingredients:
- 1 ½ cups chopped apple
- ¼ cup lemon juice
- 1 ½ tablespoons coconut oil
- 1 ½ teaspoons ground cinnamon
- Stevia to sweeten

Instructions:
1. Combine the apples, cinnamon, coconut oil and lemon juice in a small saucepan.
2. Heat over medium heat and cook for a few minutes until tender.
3. Add some stevia to sweeten if you wish.
4. Serve with puddings, porridges, crepes or just as a natural treat with some seeds for more nutrition.
5. Enjoy!

Yummy Hazelnut Treat

Servings: 4 to 6
Ingredients:
- 2 cups of raw hazelnuts
- 2 tablespoons of unsweetened raw cocoa powder
- 1 teaspoon of pure vanilla extract
- 10 drops liquid stevia

Instructions:
1. Preheat your oven to a temperature of 375°F (190 °C).
2. Spread the hazelnuts on the baking sheet and roast for about 15 minutes.
3. Place the roasted nuts into a small metal mixing bowl.
4. If you wish, cool down and remove the skins.
5. Place the hazelnuts (minus the skins) in your food processor to blend into a powder.
6. Add the cocoa powder, vanilla extract, and stevia.
7. Place in a glass container and store in a fridge.
8. Serve with puddings, porridges, or as a snack. You can also serve it with some fruit.
9. Enjoy!

Tropical Granola

Another easy way to get your morning boost is to make a huge batch of delicious granola in advance. You can easily make some to enjoy every morning all week long. You'll get a healthy source of carbohydrates from the grains used, and you'll get plenty of fats and proteins from the combination of nutritious nuts and seeds.

Serves: 4
Ingredients:
- 1 tsp coconut oil
- 2 tbsp. stevia powder
- 1 tsp ginger powder
- 1 tsp vanilla extract
- 1 cup rolled oats (cooked quinoa or amaranth also works fine)
- 1/2 tsp cinnamon
- ¼ cup almonds, soaked
- ¼ cup pumpkin seeds
- ¼ cup desiccated coconut
- ¼ cup dried dates
- Coconut yogurt to mix in
- Juice of 1 lime (optional)

Instructions:
1. Preheat the oven to 300°F.
2. Whisk the coconut oil, stevia and vanilla extract to make a syrupy mixture.
3. Mix the rolled oats with the cinnamon and pour evenly onto a baking tray. Toast the rolled oats for 10 minutes in the oven.

4. Add the almonds, pumpkin seeds and some of the desiccated coconut and mix into the semi-toasted oats.
5. Add the syrup mixture to the oats, ensuring that everything is coated well.
6. Toast the mixture for a further 20 minutes or so.
7. Add the rest of the desiccated coconut and the dried dates. Mix well and allow to cool.
8. Store in a suitable airtight container. Serve alongside some vegan-friendly yogurt such as coconut yogurt.

Alka-Berry Pancakes

This is a perfect way to incorporate the healthfulness of berries with a classic breakfast like pancakes. I like to make some on a Sunday evening so that I have something to look forward on Monday morning when I have to be up early. Besides, it's nice to get up and have a ready to grab breakfast (also great as a take-away breakfast).

Makes approximately 8 pancakes
Ingredients:
- 1 1/4 cups almond flour
- 1 tsp. stevia
- 1 1/2 tsp. baking powder
- 1 tsp. bicarbonate of soda
- Dash of Himalayan salt
- 1/2 tsp. ground nutmeg
- 1 cup coconut milk
- 1 banana, mashed
- 1 tbsp. vegan butter or coconut oil
- 1 tbsp. olive oil
- Blueberries or pomegranates or grapefruits

Instructions:
1. Combine the flour, stevia baking powder, bicarbonate of soda, nutmeg and a dash of salt in a bowl.
2. Whisk the mashed banana into the coconut milk.
3. Make a well in the middle of the flour mixture and slowly add the milk mixture, folding it in gently as you go along. Leave the mixture to sit a while.
4. Melt the vegan butter or coconut oil and the olive oil in a nonstick pan over a medium heat.

5. Ladle a small amount of the pancake batter into the pan and allow each pancake to cook one at a time. Stack them one on top of the other when cooked, making sure that you put a little vegan butter between each layer to prevent them from sticking together.
6. Serve with blueberries, or some alkaline fruits like pomegranates or grapefruits. Enjoy!

Buckwheat and Banana Porridge

This recipe is great for cold winter mornings. It will keep you full till lunch!

Servings: 2

Ingredients:

- 1 cup water
- 1 cup buckwheat grouts
- 2 big grapefruits, peeled and sliced
- Stevia to sweeten (optional)
- 1 tablespoon ground cinnamon
- 3 to 4 cups of almond milk
- 2 tablespoons natural almond butter
- Optional: 1 tablespoon of barley grass green powder

Instructions:

1. Whisk together the water and buckwheat in a medium saucepan.
2. Bring the water to boil then add buckwheat.
3. Keep cooking till the buckwheat absorbs all the water.
4. Reduce heat and add in some almond milk. Stir well.
5. Add in the rest of the ingredients except grapefruit.
6. Turn of the heat and place into cereal bowls adding some grapefruit chunks.
7. Enjoy!

Almond Paleo Style Alka-Porridge

This is a perfect and Paleo friendly alternative for those who can't tolerate grains (even healthy grains). All you need to do is to...go nuts!

Servings: 2
Ingredients:
- 1 cup chopped almonds
- 1/3 cup shredded coconut, unsweetened
- 2 tablespoons pumpkin seeds (or any other seeds of your choice)
- 2 tablespoon chia seeds
- 1 tablespoon ground flaxseed
- 1 teaspoon ground cinnamon
- 1 teaspoon almond extract
- 2 cup boiling hot water
- Coconut yoghurt or cream to serve
- Homemade sugar-free marmalade to serve (check out the next recipe)

Instructions:
1. Place all the dry ingredients (except spices) though a blender until powdered.
2. Add in some hot water and stir well.
3. Finish off by adding spices, vegan yoghurt of your choice and home-made marmalade.
4. Enjoy!

Home-Made Anti-Inflammatory Marmalade

This recipe is not only a healthy alternative to processed marmalades that are full of sugar but it's also great to help you save some money whole creating a healthy and guilt-free with anti-inflammatory properties!

Serves: 2 cups of marmalade

Ingredients:

- 1 cup pineapple chunks (small)
- 1 cup grapefruit chunks (small)
- 1 tablespoon cinnamon
- 1 tablespoon fresh grated ginger (or ginger powder)
- ½ tablespoon nutmeg
- Optional: stevia to sweeten (just a few drips will do)
- 3-4 tablespoons of coconut oil
- ¼ cup coconut milk or cream (raw, unsweetened)

Instructions:

1. Heat up coconut oil in a pan over medium heat.
2. Add the fruits and keep stirring.
3. When the fruits get slightly soft, add the spices stirring well.
4. Keep adding some coconut milk or cream to add some nice flavours and softness.
5. Keep stirring for a few minutes or until the fruits are soft.
6. Cool down and place in jars.
7. Store in a fridge for a few hours or overnight before serving.
8. Great to serve with pancakes, puddings and other treats. I also like it on raw fruits like apples.
9. Enjoy! It's really healthy!

Green Cinnamon Apple Oats

Servings: 4

Oats Ingredients:
- 2 cups of unsweetened almond milk
- 2 cups boiling water
- 2 teaspoons of vanilla extract
- 2 cups of old-fashioned oats (gluten-free)
- 2 tablespoons of chia seeds
- 1 teaspoon of ground cinnamon
- 1 tablespoon alfalfa powder or barley grass green powder
- Juice of 1 lemon
- Optional: stevia to sweeten

Apple Topping:
- 2 tablespoons of coconut oil
- 2 medium apples, cored and chopped
- Stevia (optional)
- 1 teaspoon cinnamon powder

Instructions:
1. Place oats in a cereal bowl and add in the warm water. Stir well and cover.
2. In the meantime, heat up some coconut oil in a frying pan (medium heat). Add the apples and sauté until slightly soft.
3. When done, turn off the heat and combine the apples with the oats in the cereal bowl.
4. Add almond milk, chia seeds, vanilla and alfalfa powder.
5. Sweeten with stevia if you wish.
6. Sprinkle over some lemon juice.

7. You can also serve it with some homemade marmalade from the previous recipe.
8. Enjoy!

Variations- oats can be replaced by quinoa as well as crushed nuts and seeds (for example walnuts, cashews or almonds). Experiment to your heart's content.

Spicy Pumpkin 100% Vegan Muffins

I won't lie to you; this is not the best recipe if you are pressed for time. However, it may be worth trying on a Sunday evening to make sure you have a nice take-away breakfast for the next day.

Servings: 12
Ingredients:
- 1 tablespoons of ground flaxseed
- 1/2 cup of warm water
- 2/3 cups of rice flour
- ½ cup of buckwheat flour
- ½ cup of tapioca starch
- 1 teaspoon of pumpkin pie spice
- 1 teaspoon of baking soda
- ½ teaspoon of baking powder
- ½ teaspoon of Himalayan salt
- 1 ¼ cups of pumpkin puree
- Stevia to sweeten (optional)
- ½ cup of melted coconut oil
- ¼ cup of water, cold
- 1/3 cup finely chopped almonds

To serve:

-pomegranate fruits or grapefruit slices

Instructions:
1. First, preheat your oven to a temperature of 325°F (160 Celsius)
2. In the meantime, use paper liners to line the cups of a muffin pan.

3. Combine flaxseed and the water, whisk energetically and let the mixture rest for 10 minutes.
4. In a mixing bowl, combine rice flour with buckwheat flour.
5. Add the tapioca starch, pumpkin pie spice, baking soda, baking powder and Himalayan salt.
6. Take another bowl to mix the pumpkin puree with stevia, coconut oil, water, and the flaxseed mixture.
7. Stir the dry ingredient mixture into the wet ingredient mixture. Be sure there are no lumps.
8. Fold in the almonds. Spoon the muffin batter into the muffin pan, filling each cup.
9. Bake for about 40-45 minutes. Cool down and serve with some fruit, like for example alkaline fruit (grapefruit, pomegranate etc.)

Section II

Amazingly Delicious and Nutritious Smoothies and Juices

Nice and Fresh Mint Smoothie

This smoothie is great for digestion and is full of antioxidant properties. In addition, it helps you keep hydrated and nicely refreshed. Personally, I find the mint really effective in alleviating headaches and staying energized naturally without having to resort to caffeine.

Servings: 1
Ingredients:
- Half cup of frozen or fresh blueberries
- 1 cup of fresh chopped spinach
- 1 cup of unsweetened almond milk or coconut milk
- 2 tablespoons of fresh chopped mint
- 1 teaspoon of stevia or a few banana slices

Optional (to garnish):

-a few mint leaves

-a slice of lime

Instructions:
1. Combine the spinach and almond milk in a high-speed blender.
2. Blend well until smooth and add the rest of the ingredients.
3. Blend again to make sure there are no lumps.
4. Pour your smoothie into a glass and enjoy right away.

Simple Raspberry Smoothie

Ever since I was a kid, I loved raspberries. It's one of my favourite fruits and whenever I can get it (I stick to seasonal options only) I turn them into smoothies. This one is miraculous and if you can combine it with some green powders you will create a nourishing green smoothie that is very tempting (great for green smoothie beginners). It's all about balance.

Serves: 1-2
Ingredients:
- 1 cup raspberries (you could also use blueberries)
- 1 cup almond milk or coconut milk
- Juice of 2 grapefruits
- Pinch of Himalayan salt
- Optional: 1 teaspoon of alfalfa or barley grass powder

Instructions:
1. Simply blend and serve.
2. Enjoy!

Refreshing Green Smoothie

Smoothies are always a great way to start your day and they are super quick to make. One smoothie a day will keep the doctor a way and it's better to schedule it first thing in the morning, before you get too busy.

Servings: 1 to 2
Ingredients:
- A few pineapple slices
- ½ cup baby spinach
- 1 cup coconut milk
- 6 to 8 ice cubes
- 1 teaspoon alfalfa powder or barley grass
- Juice of 2 limes

Instructions:
1. Combine the smoothie ingredients in a blender.
2. Blend until smooth and then add in the lime juice.
3. Pour your smoothie into a glass, drink and enjoy!

Sweet Cherry and Chia Smoothie

Servings: 1 to 2
Ingredients:

- ½ cup of frozen or fresh cherries
- ½ cup baby spinach
- 1 cup of almond milk
- 2 tablespoons of raw chia seeds
- Pinch ground ginger

Instructions:

1. Combine the smoothie ingredients in a blender.
2. First blend the spinach and cherries.
3. Add the milk, chia seeds and ginger.
4. Pour your finished smoothie into glasses and drink.

Spinach Green Tea Energy Smoothie

While caffeine in all its forms is not really alkaline, there is nothing wrong with an occasional cup of tea, especially green tea that is full of antioxidants and fat-burning properties. Great in a smoothie!

Servings: 2-3
Ingredients:
- 1 cup chopped baby spinach
- 1 small ripe avocado
- 1 cup brewed green tea, chilled
- Juice of 2 grapefruits
- Stevia to sweeten (optional)

Instructions:
1. Combine the smoothie ingredients in a blender and process a few times until smooth.
2. Pour your finished smoothie into glasses and drink.

Fruity Spicy Tropical Smoothie

While most fruit (especially "sugary" fruit) is not super alkaline, fruit is totally okay as a part of a balanced diet. It's also much healthier than processed carbs or sugary treats. There is no doubt about it. The spices used in this smoothie have anti-inflammatory and alkalizing properties and the green tea will give you a boost of energy.

Servings: 2-3
Ingredients:
- 1 cup blueberries
- 1 cup fresh papaya, chopped
- 1 medium banana
- A few ice cubes
- 2 cups brewed green tea, chilled
- 1 teaspoon ground turmeric
- 1 teaspoon ground ginger
- 1 teaspoon ground ginger
- Pinch cayenne pepper
- Optional: stevia

Instructions:
1. Combine the smoothie ingredients in a blender.
2. Blend well until smooth and add the spices.
3. Pour your finished smoothie into glasses and drink.
4. Enjoy!

Leafy Green Smoothie

Here is another smoothie that combines detoxifying and energizing properties. It is great to start your day feeling amazing!

Servings: 1 to 2
Ingredients:
- 1 cup of chopped kale
- 1 medium green apple, cored and chopped
- 1 stalk of celery, chopped
- ¼ cup of fresh parsley, minced
- 1 cup of fresh pomegranate or grapefruit juice
- A few ice cubes
- 1 tablespoon hemp seeds
- Stevia to sweeten (optional)

Instructions:
1. Combine the smoothie ingredients in a blender.
2. Blend well until smooth.
3. Pour your finished smoothie into a glass and drink.
4. Enjoy!

Super Alkalizing Avocado Coconut Smoothie

Servings: 1 to 2
Ingredients:
- 2 cups fresh chopped baby spinach
- 1 small chopped avocado
- ¼ cup of fresh chopped cilantro
- 1 cup chilled coconut water
- 1 tablespoon grated ginger, fresh
- ½ teaspoon ground turmeric
- Pinch cayenne

Instructions:
1. Combine the smoothie ingredients in your high-speed blender.
2. Pulse the ingredients a few times to chop them up.
3. Blend the mixture on the highest speed setting for 30 to 60 seconds.
4. Pour your finished smoothie into glasses and drink.
5. Enjoy!

Hydrating Watermelon Smoothie

This smoothie is great on a warm, summer morning, or anytime during the day. Watermelon combined with coconut water offer hydration, rejuvenation and energy.

Servings: 2-3
Ingredients:
- 1 cup frozen blueberries
- 1 cup fresh chopped watermelon
- 1 inch fresh sliced ginger
- 1 cup coconut water
- 1 tablespoon raw chia seeds
- A few ice cubes

Instructions:
1. Combine the smoothie ingredients in a blender.
2. Blend well until smooth.
3. Pour your finished smoothie into glasses and drink. Enjoy!

Ginger Protein Energy Smoothie

Servings: 1 to 2
Ingredients:
- 1 cup of chopped kale
- 1 cup pomegranates
- 1 medium carrot, diced
- 1 inch fresh grated ginger
- 1 cup coconut water
- 1 scoop hemp protein powder

Instructions:
1. Combine the smoothie ingredients in a blender.
2. Blend well until smooth.
3. Pour your finished smoothie into glasses and drink.

Peach Sweetness Smoothie

Servings: 1 to 2
Ingredients:
- 2 peaches, peeled and pitted
- 1 cup of almond milk
- 6 to 8 ice cubes
- 2 tablespoons raw hemp seeds or powder
- 1 teaspoon ground ginger
- Juice of 2 lemons

Instructions:
1. Combine the smoothie ingredients in a blender.
2. Blend until smooth, add ginger, ice cubes and hemp seeds.
3. Pour your finished smoothies into glasses and drink.
4. Enjoy!

Cucumber Melon Smoothie

I love this recipe in the summer! Honeydew melon gives it a nice taste which is great for those who are not used to drinking green smoothies.

Servings: 2
Ingredients:
- 1 cup of chopped honeydew melon
- 1 cup cucumber, diced
- 1 cup coconut water
- 1 tablespoon of fresh mint
- 1 tablespoon cilantro
- Pinch of Himalayan salt
- Juice of 1 lime
- Chia seeds (optional)

Instructions:
1. Blend the smoothie ingredients in a blender or food processor.
2. Add Himalayan salt to taste, mix well and if you wish, stir in some chia seeds for more nutrition.
3. Enjoy!

Fennel Magic Alka-Juice

Serves: 1-2

Ingredients:

- 2 cups fennel, chopped
- 2 tablespoons fennel seeds + 1 divided
- 2 cups spinach
- 2 cups carrot slices
- 1 pear, peeled and sliced
- ½ cup lemon juice
- Ice cubes

Instructions:

1. Wash all ingredients well. Clean and chop.
2. Add all ingredients (fennel, spinach, carrots, pear) through juicer.
3. Mix in some lemon juice. Place in a tall glass
4. Serve with a sprinkling of fennel seeds on top and it is best served chilled.
5. Ice cubes, and ginger ice cubes work great with this juice.
6. Enjoy!

Sweet Grapefruit Easy Mix

Pressed for time and want to alkalize? This recipe is super easy and full of alkalinity!

Serves: 1-2

Ingredients:

- 2 grapefruits
- 1 cup coconut water
- 1 cup almond milk
- ½ lemon
- 1 teaspoon powdered ginger
- ¼ cup warm water (not boiling)

Instructions:

1. Combine the powdered ginger and warm water until dissolved.
2. Add the lemon and grapefruit juice.
3. Add the coconut water and almond milk.
4. Add ice cubes or ginger ice cubes.
5. Enjoy!

Kukicha Smoothie

Ever heard of kukicha? If not, make sure you put it on your alkaline shopping list. If yes, I hope the following recipe will help you come up with more ideas on your alkaline journey!

Serves: 2
Ingredients:
- 1 cup kukicha tea
- 1 cup coconut milk
- ½ cup spinach
- 1 banana
- 1 inch ginger
- A green apple
- ¼ cup almonds (soaked in water for 8 hours or more)
- Optional: juice of 1 lemon

Instructions:
1. Blend all the ingredients until smooth.
2. For more alkalinity, add some lemon juice.
3. Stir well, serve, and enjoy!

Nice'n Fresh Smoothie

Soy sprouts and alfalfa sprouts are great, not only in your salads and soups, but also in your smoothies. When combined with other healthy and alkalizing ingredients, they create amazing alkaline balance and taste.

Serves: 2
Ingredients:
- 2 cups almond milk (unsweetened)
- ½ cup soy sprouts
- ½ cup alfalfa sprouts
- 1 inch ginger
- ½ an avocado
- 1 green apple
- 1 tablespoon avocado oil or coconut oil
- stevia to sweeten (optional)

Instructions:
1. Combine all the ingredients, except for oils, in a blender.
2. Blend until smooth.
3. Add some coconut oil or avocado oil. If you wish, sweeten with some stevia.
4. Enjoy!

Wake Up Maca Juice

Green, alkaline juices are natural energy boosters; however, by adding some maca powder, we can really take it to the next level!

Servings: 2-3
Ingredients:
- 1/2 cup water cress
- 3 big tomatoes
- A few fennel slices
- ½ inch ginger
- ½ cup parsley
- Juice of 1 lemon
- ½ teaspoon of maca powder
- 1 tablespoon olive oil or avocado oil

Procedure:
1. Wash and chop all the veggies.
2. Place through a juicer.
3. Place the juice in a tall glass and add some maca powder and lemon juice.
4. Add some olive or avocado oil for better absorption.

Additional Information:
Maca
This natural supplement is rich in Vitamin C, B, and E, as well as zinc, iron, calcium, magnesium, phosphorus, and amino acids. It has hormone balancing properties and acts as an aphrodisiac, both for men and women. As far as female health is concerned, maca can help alleviate menstrual cramps, as well as menopause issues (mood swings, depression, and anxiety).

Contraindications: avoid maca if pregnant or lactating. If on medication or suffering from any serious health problems, remember to contact your doctor first.

When trying maca for the first time, use no more than ½ teaspoon a day and go from there. The recommended maximum intake is actually about 1 teaspoon a day. However, remember that maca acts as a stimulant. Listen to your body; sometimes less is better.

Boost Your Metabolism Juice

This recipe offers a unique taste, pH balancing properties, metabolism boosting properties, and is also great for your skin.

Servings: 1-2
Ingredients:
- 1 cup fresh spinach
- 1 large grapefruit, juiced
- 1 carrot, small
- 2 celery stalks
- 1 beet
- ½ teaspoon cinnamon
- 1/2 inch of fresh stem ginger
- ¼ cup fresh mint leaves
- 1 tablespoon chia seeds

Procedure:
1. Wash the spinach, mint, grapefruit, carrot, celery stalks, and beet.
2. Chop the spinach, carrot (no need to peel if organic), celery, and beet.
3. Place through a juicer. While the juicer is working, you may juice the grapefruit (I use a simple lemon squeezer).
4. Mix the fresh veggie juice with grapefruit juice.
5. Add some chia seeds and stir well.
6. Drink immediately.
7. Enjoy!

Purple Energy Detox Juice

Beet root is extremely good for cleansing the liver. While I do agree it might not be the best juice for beginners, I can also tell you it's worth getting used to it. The juice is jam-packed with minerals and great for shedding unwanted pounds, not to mention higher energy levels! Lemon and lime juice add more flavor to this juice and make it a great, refreshing drink for any time of the day.

Servings: 1-2
Ingredients:
- 2 celery stalks
- 2 medium cucumbers
- ¼ cup parsley
- ¼ cup mint
- 1 beet root
- 1 lemon, juiced
- 1 lime, juiced
- 1 tsp olive oil
- Pinch of Himalayan salt

Procedure:
1. Wash and chop all the ingredients.
2. Place celery, cucumbers, parsley, mint and beet root through a juicer.
3. When ready, place the juice in a juice glass or another utensil of your choice and stir in some lemon and lime juice, as well as Himalayan salt and a bit of olive oil (or any other quality cold-pressed oil) of your choice. Oils help your body with nutrient absorption. Enjoy!

SECTION III Hunger Satisfying Alkaline Recipes

Chilled Spicy Avocado Soup

I know what you are thinking… "Soup… for breakfast?" Well, everything is possible in the alkaline world. This recipe is perfect if you want to increase your energy levels; it's raw and 100% alkaline! You can even prepare more and save it in your fridge to have a healthy, energizing elixir to sip on during the day. It's a great recipe if you wish to reduce inflammation, detoxify and start losing weight.

Servings: 2
Ingredients:
- 2 large avocados, pitted and chopped
- 2 cucumbers, peeled and diced
- 1/2 cup coconut yogurt or coconut cream
- 2 tablespoons of chopped chives
- 2 tablespoons of cilantro
- 1 tablespoon of fresh lime juice
- 1 teaspoon of Himalayan salt
- ½ small jalapeno, seeded and minced
- Pinch of cayenne pepper or black pepper to taste (curry is also an option)
- 1 teaspoon of minced ginger
- 1/2 teaspoon of minced garlic

Instructions:
1. Place all the ingredients (except spices) in a food processor and blend until smooth.
2. Add chives, cilantro, lime juice. Himalaya salt, jalapeno, pepper, ginger and garlic

3. You can add in some water if you don't like thick consistency.
4. Pour the soup into a serving bowl and chill it for at least an hour until cold.
5. Another option is to have this soup slightly warm.
6. Enjoy!

Thai Tofu and Vegetable Curry

I know what you're thinking, "Curry for breakfast?" Well, why not? It's a great option if you wake up hungry or are looking for a filling breakfast recipe after a morning workout. This recipe is fantastic on a cold, winter morning and relatively quick to make.

Servings: 2
Ingredients:
- 1 cup of vegetable broth (low sodium)
- 1 cup of coconut milk
- ½ tablespoon of Thai red curry paste
- ¼ teaspoon ground ginger
- Himalayan salt to taste
- 1 cup red bell pepper
- Half cup green beans, trimmed
- 1 cup of chopped carrots
- 1 medium sweet potato, peeled and chopped
- ½ cup of diced tofu
- 1 tablespoon of fresh lime juice
- 1 tablespoons of fresh chopped basil

Instructions:
1. Combine the vegetable broth, coconut milk, ginger and salt and curry paste in a medium saucepan.
2. Bring to a boil.
3. Stir in red bell pepper, beans, carrots and sweet potato.
4. Simmer for 5 minutes until just turning tender.
5. Stir in the tofu and cook for a few minutes more.
6. Finally, add in some lime juice, basil, salt and pepper to taste.
7. Serve hot. Enjoy!

Breakfast Kale Soup

I know that many people can be put off by the name of this recipe, but don't reject it before you have tried it. Kale is miraculous and this soup will help keep you warm and energized on cold winter mornings. It can also be served chilled as a natural tool to feed your body with nutrients.

Serves: 2
Ingredients:
- 1 small onion, chopped
- 3 cloves garlic, minced
- 2 celery stalks, diced
- 2 tablespoons red wine
- 4 tablespoons olive oil or coconut oil
- 4 cups vegetable stock
- 1 teaspoon Himalayan salt
- ¼ teaspoon black pepper
- ¼ teaspoon dried basil (or 1 tsp fresh)
- 1 can cooked chickpeas, rinsed and drained
- 1 cup kale no stems, ale, cut into strips

Instructions:
1. First, sauté celery, garlic and onion in the oil for 3-4 minutes (medium heat)
2. Add veggie stock as well as basil, chickpeas, salt and pepper.
3. Bring to a boil (covered).Reduce heat and simmer for about 15 minutes on medium heat.
4. Blend the mixture.
5. Once blended, pour the mixture back into the pot, adding the kale and simmering for 10 minutes. Serve hot.

Awesome Alkaline Tacos

Great breakfast idea if you wake up feeling hungry or are not in the mood for smoothies or porridges.

Serves: 2-4
Ingredients:
- 4 gluten-free tortillas
- 1 cooked sweet potato
- Green beans
- Salad greens (kale, spinach, lettuce, chard, arugula - it's up to you)
- 1 avocado, peeled, pitted and sliced
- Half cup black beans, cooked
- Spices to taste (cumin, chili powder, garlic powder, onion powder and cayenne pepper are my favorite)

Instructions:
1. If you wish, warm the tortillas in the oven or over the stove. Careful not to burn them. I suggest you heat them on a low flame for 10 seconds on each side.
2. Blend the sweet potato with the spices.
3. Spread the mixture across the center of each tortilla. Add beans, avocado and greens on top.
4. Serve with some fresh tomato and tomato slices for more alkaline properties.
5. Enjoy!

Energizing Breakfast Potatoes Brunch

This is a fantastic brunch recipe for those who are starving!

Serves: 2
Ingredients:
- 2 tablespoons olive oil
- 2 cups sweet potatoes
- 1 large onion
- 2 tablespoons capers
- Vegan sour cream
- 1 Tablespoon Dijon mustard
- Salt and pepper to taste
- Mixed greens for side salad

Instructions:
1. Wash, peel and chop potatoes.
2. Take a medium-size skillet and heat up the olive oil, adding potatoes and scallions (medium-heat)
3. Sautee adding some water until potatoes are soft. Keep stirring.
4. Combine all remaining ingredients in a bowl, except the greens. Place on a plate and pour sour cream mixture on top.
5. Serve with green leafy greens.
6. Enjoy!

Red Pepper Hummus

This hummus is great with some raw veggies, gluten free wraps or homemade bread!

Servings: 10 to 12
Ingredients:
- 1.5 cup chickpeas, cooked, rinsed and drained
- 1 cup of roasted red peppers, chopped
- 2 cloves minced garlic
- 1/4 jalapeno, seeded and minced
- Himalayan salt and black pepper to taste
- 4 tablespoons olive oil
- Water, as needed

Instructions:
1. Combine the chickpeas, roasted red pepper, garlic and jalapeno in a food processor.
2. Blend well until smooth.
3. Season with salt and pepper to taste.
4. Add in the oil and water for desired consistency.
5. Serve with sliced veggies, in wraps and sandwiches.
6. Enjoy!

Baked Spicy Kale Chips

Servings: 4 to 6
Ingredients:

- 3 cups of kale leaves
- Olive oil or coconut oil
- Himalayan salt, black pepper, curry powder (or your favourite spices), to taste

Instructions:

1. Preheat the oven to 220°F and line two rimmed baking sheets with parchment paper.
2. Massage the kale leaves in oil and spread them on baking sheets in a single layer.
3. Sprinkle liberally with spices and add salt.
4. Bake for 40 minutes, carefully flipping the sides. Kale is easy to burn to keep an eye on the oven.
5. Turn off the oven and let the kale cool until crisp.
6. Enjoy!

Serve with hummus or vegetable dips. You can also take it as a take away breakfast or snack.

Simple Bean Breakfast

Quick and Easy!
Serves: 2
Ingredients:

- 1 can white haricot beans
- 4 spring onions (early picked, red onion) chopped
- 6 grape tomatoes halved or quartered
- 2 tablespoons fresh chopped basil
- 2 cups fresh spinach
- 3 cloves chopped garlic
- 1 avocado (peeled and pitted)
- ½ squeezed lemon
- Coconut/olive oil
- Himalayan salt/black pepper
- Leafy greens (side salad) of your choice - enough for 2 people

Preparation:

1. Heat about 3 tablespoons water in a frying pan and steam fry chopped garlic (about one minutes.).
2. Add tomatoes, beans and onions, until soft.
3. Put in the basil and spinach. Allow to wilt, and then sprinkle with pepper and salt.
4. Slice the avocado. Put the bean mix over the greens and top with avocado. Drizzle olive oil over the top and finish with a squeeze of lemon.
5. Enjoy!

Alkaline Green Wraps

Do you know the feeling when you wake up hungry? Well, the alkaline solution is simple - go for alkaline, gluten free wraps!

Serves: 1
Ingredients:
- 2 gluten-free, yeast-free wraps
- 1 cup of radish, chopped
- 2 garlic cloves, chopped
- ½ cup of freshly made hummus or tahini
- 1 avocado, sliced
- 1 cucumber, peeled and diced

Preparation (2 simple steps for busy people!):

1. Mix all the ingredients in a salad bowl. Add olive oil, lemon juice, tahini (or hummus) and Himalayan salt.
2. Place the filling in each wrap, roll up and serve!
3. Enjoy! Alkaline wraps are real life savers. They keep you full, alkalize your body and mind, and you don't feel like you are missing something...

Raw Alkaline Breakfast

Have you ever considered having delicious alkaline salads first thing in the morning? If not, why not? This recipe is great for hot summers! Raw foods and alkalinity go hand in hand!

Serves: 1

Ingredients:
- Half avocado
- ½ cup of alfalfa sprouts
- 2 tomatoes
- 1 cucumber
- 2 onion rings, minced
- Half garlic clove, minced
- 1 tablespoon avocado oil
- ¼ cup of raw almonds
- Himalayan salt and black pepper to taste
- Optional: ¼ cup cooked lentils or chickpeas (great in the winter)
- Juice of half a lemon

Preparation:
1. Mix all the veggies in a salad bowl.
2. Drizzle over some avocado oil, lemon juice and season with Himalayan salt and black pepper.
3. Enjoy!

Afterword- Stay Alkaline and Don't Worry Too Much!

The aim of this recipe book was to show you how you can adapt to a clean alkaline diet. This alkaline inspired cuisine allows you to still eat mouth-watering, healthy, wholesome meals that will enable you to live life to the fullest without feeling deprived.

I really hope you'll continue to get a lot of use out of this book as you progress with your alkaline diet lifestyle returning again and again to your favourite recipes. Here's wishing you all the best in your health and wellness journey!

If you enjoyed my book, it would be greatly appreciated if you left a review so others can receive the same benefits you have. Your review can help other people take this important step to take care of their health and inspire them to start a new chapter in their lives. At the same time, you can help me serve you and all my other readers even more.

I'd be thrilled to hear from you. I would love to know your top 3 recipes! Or at least your favourite recipe or section. As long as I know what you like, I can create more amazing recipes and tips that will help you on your journey.

I know you are busy and I would like to thank you in advance for considering taking a couple of minutes to review this book. Even one sentence will do. Thanks!

Your comments are very important to me.

Your 3 FREE eBooks + Alkaline Wellness Newsletter

Don't forget to download your free eBooks.
They are waiting for you at:
www.holisticwellnessproject.com/alkaline

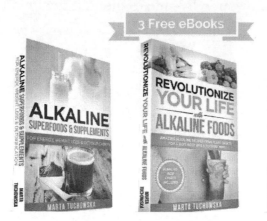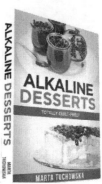

Let Me Help You

If you have any questions, doubts, or you find my instructions confusing and need more guidance, please e-mail me. I am here to help. Don't be shy. I am also looking for feedback. If you have any suggestions that can help me improve my work, please let me know and I will take an immediate action to serve you better in the next editions.

info@holisticwellnessproject.com

More Alkaline & Wellness Books by Marta:

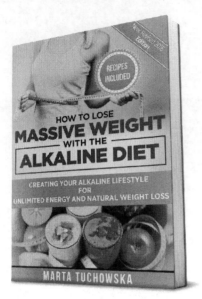

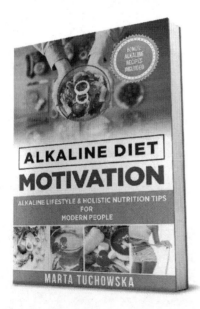

You will find them + many more at:
www.holisticwellnessproject.com/books

FINALLY- LET'S KEEP IN TOUCH:

www.instagram.com/Marta_Wellness

www.facebook.com/HolisticWellnessProject

www.twitter.com/Marta_Wellness

www.pinterest.com/martaWellness/

I wish you wellness, health, and success in whatever it is that you want to accomplish.
With lots of LOVE and positive energy,

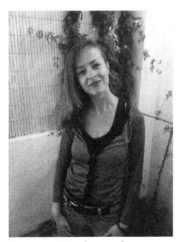

Marta Tuchowska

Made in the USA
Lexington, KY
07 September 2017